Mediterranean Diet Cookbook

Delicious And Affordable Recipes To Lose
Weight Enjoying Your Favorite Foods

Chef Angela Doria

Additionally, the information in the following pages is intended only for informational purposes and should thus be thought of as universal. As befitting its nature, it is presented without assurance regarding its prolonged validity or interim quality. Trademarks that are mentioned are done without written consent and can in no way be considered an endorsement from the trademark holder.

Table of Contents

—

Introduction

"Mediterranean diet" is a common term and inspired by the eating habits of Spain, Greece, and Italy in the 1960s. This diet highlights the whole grain, seafood, vegetable, fruits, low intake of dairy product such as yogurt and cheese, olive oil, sweets, and red meats. This diet is linked with various health benefits, such as it lowers the risk of cancer, type-2 diabetes, obesity, and cognitive diseases. This diet offers a cuisine rich in taste, color, and aroma. A perfect Mediterranean diet does not offer canola oil, soybeans or any other unhealthy oil. It is characterized by the balanced use of food items with a high number of fibers, unsaturated fats, and antioxidant. This magical diet has magical recipes that have a delicious and mouthwatering taste.

My big wish is that "The Mediterranean diet cookbook will inspire you to spend good time in your kitchen. This cookbook is full of all kinds of meals that you want to eat. You will find yummy recipes based on different chapters such as smoothies/breakfast, salad, pasta, rice and grain, seafood and fish, vegetables, meat, poultry, egg recipes, vegetarian, bread and pizza, snacks, and dessert and fruit. All food fits in your diet and best for your health.

In addition, this cookbook will inspire to keep healthy always and eat good food. When you follow this diet, you will live a happier, healthier, and more fulfilling life. All recipes are full of essential nutrients.

In Mediterranean diet:
Eat: Extra-virgin olive oil, seafood, fish, spices, herbs, breads, whole grains, potatoes, legumes, seeds, nuts, vegetable and fruits.
Eat rarely: Red meat
Eat in moderation: Yogurt, cheese, eggs, and poultry
Do not eat: Refined oil, refined grains, processed meat, added sugar, beverages, sugar-sweetened, and highly processed foods.
Avoid food:
Added sugar – table sugar, ice cream, candies, and soda
Tran's fat – It is found in Margarine and many other processed foods.
Refined grains – pasta prepared with refined wheat and white bread
Refined oil – cottonseed oil, canola oil, and soybean oil
Processed meat – hot dogs and processed sausages
High processed foods – low fat food
Food to eat:
Vegetable – cucumbers, Brussels sprouts, cauliflower, onion, carrots, spinach, kale, broccoli, and tomatoes
Fruits – peach, melon, figs, dates, strawberries, grapes, oranges, pears, apples, and bananas
Seeds and nuts – pumpkin seeds, sunflower seeds, cashews, hazelnuts, walnuts, macadamia nuts, and almonds
Tubers – yams, turnips, potatoes, and sweet potatoes
Legumes – chickpeas, peanuts, pulses, lentils, peas, and beans
Fish and seafood – mussels, crab, clams, oyster, shrimp, mackerel, tuna, trout, sardine, and salmon
Whole grains – pasta, bread, whole-grain, whole wheat, buckwheat, corn, barley, rye, brown rice, and whole oats
Poultry – turkey, duck, and chicken
Eggs – duck eggs, quail, and chicken
Herbs and spices – pepper, cinnamon, nutmeg, sage, rosemary, mint, basil, and garlic
Dairy – Greek yogurt, cheese, Greek yogurt
Healthy fats – avocado oil, olive oil, and Extra-virgin olive
What to drink:

—

Water is the best ingredients for the Mediterranean diet. Tea and Coffee are also acceptable in this diet but avoid sugar-sweetened beverages – Moderate about red wine – one glass per day.

Simple shopping list for Mediterranean diet:

Fruits – grapes, oranges, bananas, and apples

Vegetable – garlic, kale, spinach, broccoli, onion, and carrots

Berries – blueberries and strawberries

Legumes – beans, pulses, and lentils

Grains – whole-grain pasta and whole-grain bread

Seeds – pumpkin seeds and sunflower seeds

Nuts – cashews, walnuts, and almonds

Fish and seafood – trout, mackerel, sardines, and salmon

Condiments – cinnamon, turmeric, pepper, and sea salt

Greek yogurt, cheese, potatoes, sweet potatoes, chicken, olives, eggs, Extra-virgin olive oil

Health benefits for the Mediterranean diet:

The Mediterranean diet consists of enormous quantities of vegetables, fruits, olive oil, fish, and nuts and reduces physical and mental health problems.

It prevents heart disease – Following the Mediterranean diet limits intake of red meat, processed food, refined bread, and drinking red wine instead of hard liquor and these all factors help prevent stroke and heart diseases.

Reduced the risk of Alzheimer's – Research suggests that the Mediterranean diet improves blood sugar level, cholesterol, and blood vessel health.

Increase longevity – This diet increases age because it reduces the risk of cancer and heart diseases.

Halve the risk of Parkinson disease – In this diet, there is a high level of antioxidant, and it can prevent cells from damaging, and it halves the risk of Parkinson's disease.

It protects from type-2 diabetes – This diet is rich in fiber which digests gradually.

Breakfast Chia Yogurt Pudding

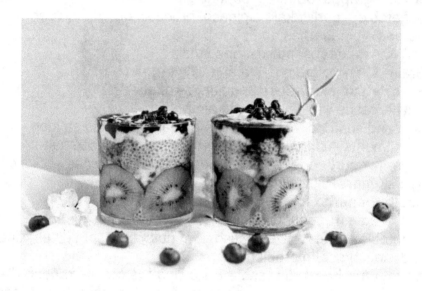

Preparation time:	Additional time:	Servings:
10 minutes	1 hour 15 minutes	4

Ingredients:

- One cup unsweetened soy milk
- One cup Greek yogurt
- Two tablespoons hulled hemp seeds
- Two tablespoons ground flax seeds
- One tablespoon honey
- One teaspoon ground cinnamon
- One teaspoon vanilla extract
- 2/3 cup chia seeds

Instructions:

- First, whisk Greek yogurt and soy milk into the big sealable container.
- Add vanilla extract, cinnamon, honey, flax seeds, and hemp seeds into the yogurt mixture.
- Add chia seeds into the yogurt mixture. Cover with lid. Place into the fridge for fifteen minutes. Stir well.

Additional Tip:

- Sprinkle with chia seeds.

Nutrition:

Calories;263,Protein; 10.4, Carbohydrates; 21.1g, Fat; 15.9g, Cholesterol; 11.3mg, Sodium; 68.7mg.

Delicious Poached Eggs Caprese

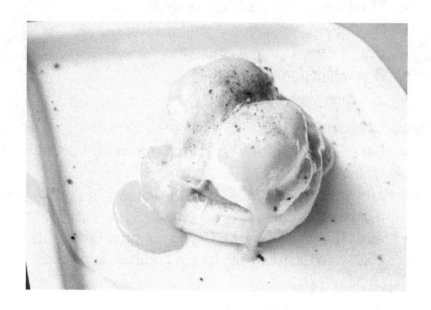

Preparation time:	Cooking time:	Servings:
10 minutes	10 minutes	2

Ingredients:

- One tablespoon distilled white vinegar
- Two teaspoons salt
- Four eggs
- Two English muffin – split
- One-ounce mozzarella cheese
- One tomato – thickly sliced
- Four teaspoons pesto
- Salt – to taste

Instructions:

- Add water into the saucepan and boil over a high flame. Decrease the speed of the flame to medium-low. Add in two tsp salt and vinegar.
- Add a slice of mozzarella cheese and tomato to the English muffin half. Place into the toaster oven and toast for five minutes until cheese is melted.
- Break an egg into the bowl. Hold the bowl above the surface of the water and then slip the egg into the simmered water. Poach the eggs for three minutes until the white part gets firm and the yolk part gets thick.
- Remove the eggs from the water using a slotted spoon and place them on the kitchen towel.
- Assemble: Add a poached egg to the English muffin.
- Add one tsp of pesto sauce to each egg.

Additional Tip:

- Sprinkle with salt.

Nutrition:

Calories;482, Protein; 33.3g, Carbohydrates; 31.7g, Fat; 24.9g, Cholesterol; 411.6mg, Sodium; 3092.7mg.

Breakfast Eggs and Greens Dish

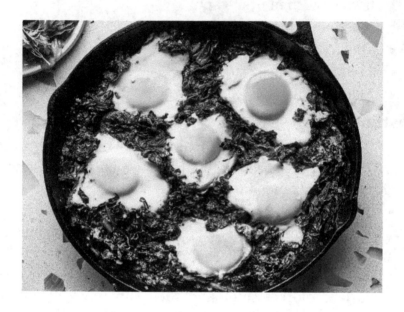

Preparation time: 10 minutes	Cooking time: 10 minutes	Servings: 2

Ingredients:

- One tablespoon olive oil
- Two cups rainbow chard – chopped, stemmed
- One cup fresh spinach
- Half cup arugula
- Two cloves garlic – minced
- Four eggs – beaten
- Half cup shredded Cheddar cheese
- Salt and ground black pepper – to taste

Instructions:

- Add oil into the skillet and cook over a medium-high flame.
- Add arugula, spinach, and chard and cook for three minutes.
- Add garlic and cook for two minutes until fragrant.
- Combine the cheese and eggs into the bowl. Add in chard mixture.
- Cover with lid. Cook for five to seven minutes – season with pepper and salt.

Additional Tip:

- Serve with tea.

Nutrition:

Calories; 333, Protein; 21g, Carbohydrates; 4.2g, Fat; 26.2g, Cholesterol; 401.7mg, Sodium; 483.5mg.

Breakfast Pita Pizza

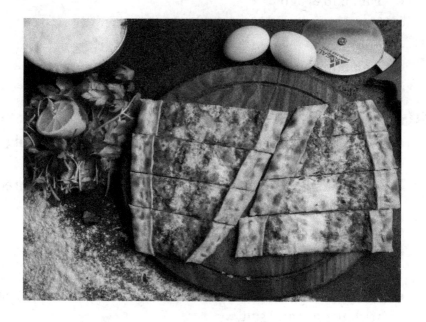

Preparation time:	Cooking time:	Servings:
25 minutes	30 minutes	2

Ingredients:

- Four slices bacon
- ¼ onion – chopped
- Two tablespoons extra-virgin olive oil
- Four eggs – beaten
- Two tablespoons pesto
- Two pita bread rounds
- Half tomato – chopped
- ¼ cup fresh mushrooms – chopped
- Half cup spinach – chopped
- Half cup shredded Cheddar cheese
- One avocado – peeled, pitted, and sliced

Instructions:

- Preheat the oven to 350 degrees Fahrenheit.
- Line a baking sheet with parchment paper.
- Add bacon into the big skillet and cook over a medium-high flame for ten minutes. Drain it onto the paper towels.
- Add the onion to another skillet and cook for five minutes until soft and translucent. Remove and keep it aside.
- Add olive oil into the skillet and add in eggs and cook for three to five minutes until set.
- Place pita bread on the lined baking sheet. Scatter pesto over the pita.
- Top with spinach, mushrooms, tomato, scrambled egg, and bacon.
- Sprinkle with cheddar cheese.
- Place into the oven and bake for ten minutes.

Additional Tip:

- Garnish with avocado slice.

Nutrition:

Calories; 873kcal, Protein; 36.8g, Carbohydrates; 43.5g,Fat; 62.9g, Cholesterol; 426.5mg, Sodium; 1134.6mg.

Tasty Caprese on Toast

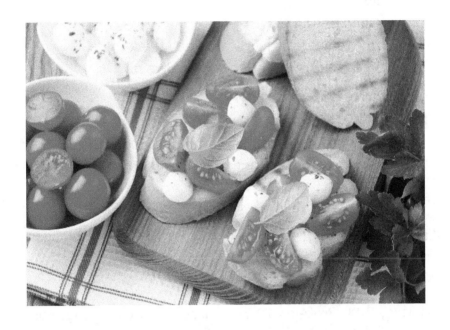

Preparation time:	Cooking time:	Servings:
15 minutes	5 minutes	14

Ingredients:

- Fourteen slices sourdough bread
- Two cloves garlic – peeled
- One pound fresh mozzarella cheese – sliced 1/4-inch thick
- 1/3 cup fresh basil leaves
- Three tomatoes – sliced 1/4-inch thick
- Three tablespoons extra-virgin olive oil
- Salt and ground black pepper – to taste

Instructions:

- First, toast bread slice and rub one side with garlic. Add one slice of tomato, one to two basil leaves, and one slice of mozzarella cheese on the slice of toast.
- Drizzle with olive oil.

Additional Tip:

- Season with black pepper and salt.

Nutrition:

Calories; 204, Protein; 10.5g, Carbohydrates; 16.5g, Fat; 10.7g, Cholesterol; 25.6mg, Sodium; 367.9mg.

Mediterranean Breakfast Quinoa

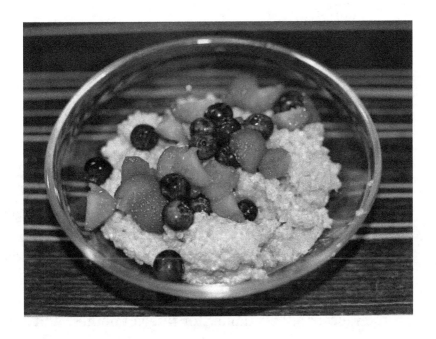

Preparation time:	Cooking time:	Servings:
10 minutes	15 minutes	4

Ingredients:

- ¼ cup raw almonds – chopped
- One teaspoon ground cinnamon
- One cup quinoa
- Two cups milk
- One teaspoon sea salt
- One teaspoon vanilla extract
- Two tablespoons honey
- Two dried pitted dates – chopped
- Five dried apricots – chopped

Instructions:

- Add almonds into the skillet and toast over a medium flame for three to five minutes until golden. Keep it aside.
- Add quinoa and cinnamon into the saucepan and cook over a medium flame.
- Add sea salt and milk into the saucepan and stir and boil the mixture.
- Decrease the speed of the flame to low. Cover the lid on the saucepan. Let simmer for fifteen minutes. Add half of the almonds, apricots, dates, honey, and vanilla into the quinoa mixture.

Additional Tip:

- Top with remaining almonds.

Nutrition:

Calories; 327, Protein; 11.5g, Carbohydrates; 53.9g, Fat; 7.9g, Cholesterol; 9.8mg, Sodium; 500.9mg.

Special Eggs Florentine

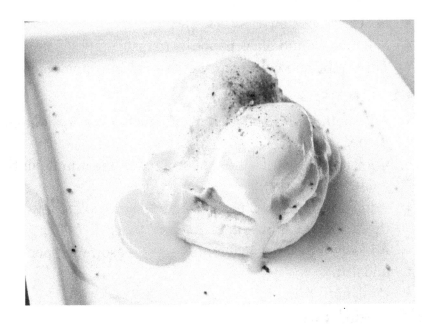

Preparation time:	Cooking time:	Servings:
10 minutes	10 minutes	3

Ingredients:
- Two tablespoons butter
- Half cup mushrooms – sliced
- Two cloves garlic – minced
- 10 ounce fresh spinach
- Six eggs – beaten
- Salt and ground black pepper – to taste
- Three tablespoons cream cheese – cut into small pieces

Instructions:
- Add butter into the skillet and melt over a medium flame.
- Cook and stir garlic and mushroom for one minute until golden and fragrant.
- Add spinach to mushroom mixture and cook for two to three minutes until wilted.
- Add egg into the spinach mixture – season with pepper and salt.
- Cook until firm.

Additional Tip:
Sprinkle With Cream Cheese And Cook For Five Minutes. Serve! Calories; 279, Protein; 15.7g, Carbohydrates; 4.1g, Fat; 22.9g, Cholesterol; 408.3mg, Sodium; 276mg.

Breakfast Shakshuka

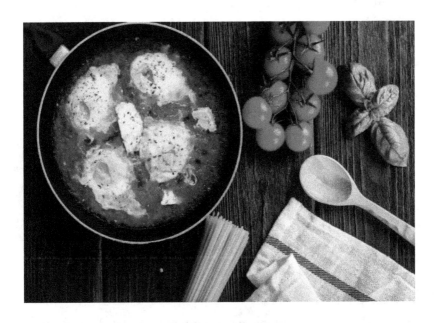

Preparation time:	Cooking time:	Servings:
15 minutes	30 minutes	6

Ingredients:

- Two tablespoons olive oil
- One onion – diced
- Half cup sliced fresh mushrooms
- One teaspoon salt
- One cup red bell pepper – diced
- One jalapeno pepper – seeded and sliced
- One teaspoon cumin
- Half teaspoon paprika
- Half teaspoon ground turmeric
- Half teaspoon freshly ground black pepper
- ¼ teaspoon cayenne pepper
- 28-ounce crushed tomatoes
- Half cup water
- Six eggs
- Two tablespoons crumbled feta cheese
- Two tablespoons fresh parsley – chopped

Instructions:

- Add olive oil into the heavy skillet and cook over a medium-high flame.
- Add mushrooms and onion and sprinkle with salt.
- Cook for ten minutes until all liquid is released.
- Add in jalapeno pepper and bell pepper and cook for five minutes – season with cayenne, black pepper, turmeric, paprika, and cumin.
- Cook for one minute. Add in water and crushed tomatoes.
- Turn the heat to medium and boil for fifteen to twenty minutes until soft.
- Add more water if the sauce gets too thick. Next, make a hole into the sauce for each egg using a big spoon.

- Break an egg into the ramekin, add to each, and repeat with remaining eggs – season with pepper and salt.
- Cover with lid and cook until the desired doneness.

Additional Tip:

- Top with fresh parsley and feta cheese.

Nutrition:

Calories; 185, Protein; 9.9g, Carbohydrates; 14.9g, Fat; 10.8g,Cholesterol; 188.8mg,Sodium; 669.8mg.

Breakfast Quinoa Cereal

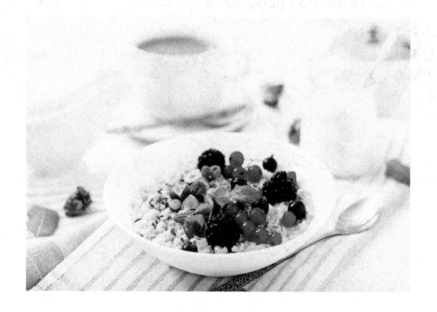

Preparation time:	Cooking time:	Servings:
5 minutes	16 minutes	4

Ingredients:

- Two cups water
- One cup quinoa – rinsed
- Half cup dried apricots – chopped
- Half cup slivered almonds
- 1/3 cup flax seeds
- One teaspoon ground cinnamon
- Half teaspoon ground nutmeg

Instructions:

- Add quinoa and water into the saucepan and cook over a medium flame. Boil it.
- Decrease the speed of the flame and simmer for eight to twelve minutes.
- Add in nutmeg, cinnamon, flax seeds, almonds, and apricots and cook for two to three minutes until tender.

Additional Tip:

- Sprinkle with nutmeg.

Nutrition:

Calories; 350, Protein; 11.8g,Carbohydrates; 44.5g,Fat; 15.1g,Sodium; 12.8mg.

Healthy Breakfast Sandwich

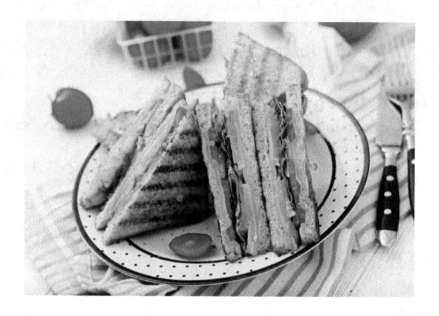

Preparation time:	Cooking time:	Servings:
5 minutes	5 minutes	2

Ingredients:

- ¾ cup liquid egg whites
- Two whole-wheat English muffins – split
- Half cup baby spinach leaves
- Two slices fresh tomato

Instructions:

- Add egg whites into the non-stick skillet and cook over a medium flame for four minutes.
- Next, toast the English muffins. Split cooked egg whites among two muffins and top with spinach, one tomato slice, and muffin tops.

Additional Tip:

- Serve with Mediterranean smoothie.

Nutrition:

Calories; 186, Protein; 16.3g,Carbohydrates; 28.8g,Fat; 1.5g, Sodium; 474mg.

Spinach Feta Egg Wrap

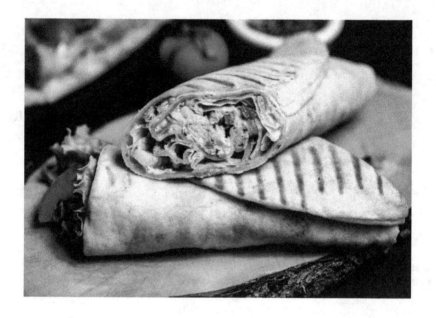

Preparation time:	Cooking time:	Servings:
10 minutes	5 minutes	1

Ingredients:

- One whole-wheat tortilla
- 1 ½ teaspoons olive oil
- One cup baby spinach leaves – chopped
- One sun-dried tomato – chopped
- Two eggs – beaten
- 1/3 cup feta cheese
- One tomato – diced

Instructions:

- First, warm the tortilla into the big skillet over a medium flame.
- Add olive oil to another skillet and melt over a medium-high flame.
- Add tomato and spinach in hot oil and cook until wilted for one minute.
- Add eggs and cook for two minutes until set. Sprinkle with feta cheese and cook for one minute.
- Transfer the egg mixture to the warm tortilla into the big skillet. Top with diced tomato and roll the tortilla and leave it in the skillet for half a minute until it holds its shape.

Additional Tip:

- Serve with butter.

Nutrition:

Calories; 704, Protein; 36.6g, Carbohydrates; 78g, Fat; 36.8g, Cholesterol; 446.8mg, Sodium; 1721.5mg.

Breakfast Zucchini with Egg

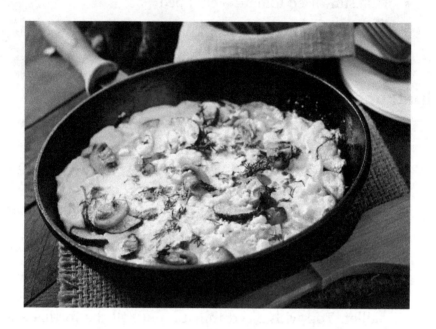

Preparation time: 5 minutes	cooking time: 15 minutes	Servings: 2

Ingredients:

- 1 ½ tablespoons olive oil
- Two zucchini – cut into large chunks
- Salt and ground black pepper – to taste
- Two eggs
- One teaspoon water

Instructions:

- Add oil into the skillet and cook over a medium-high flame. Add zucchini and cook for ten minutes until tender – season with black pepper and salt.
- Add eggs into the bowl and beat well. Add water and mix well.
- Add eggs over the zucchini and cook for five minutes until no longer runny.

Additional Tip:

- Season with black pepper and salt.

Nutrition:

Calories; 213, Protein; 10.2g, Carbohydrates; 11.2g, Fat; 15.7g, Cholesterol; 186mg,Sodium; 180mg.

Baked Eggs in Avocado

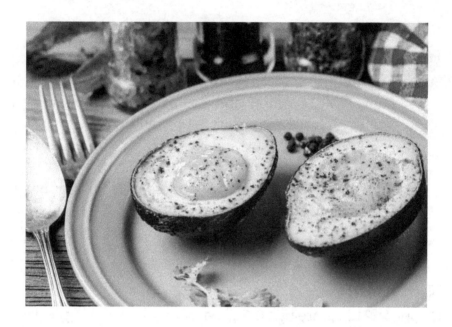

Preparation time: 10 minutes	Cooking time: 15 minutes	Servings: 2

Ingredients:

- Two eggs
- One avocado – halved and pitted
- Two slices cooked bacon – crumbled
- Two teaspoons chopped fresh chives
- One pinch dried parsley
- One pinch sea salt and ground black pepper – to taste

Instructions:

- Preheat the oven to 425 degrees Fahrenheit.
- Next, break the eggs into the bowl. Place avocado halves on the baking dish. Add one egg yolk into the avocado hole until full. Repeat with remaining avocado, egg whites, and egg yolk – season with pepper, sea salt, fresh parsley, and chives.
- Place the baking dish into the oven and bake for fifteen minutes and sprinkle with bacon.
- Serve and enjoy!

Additional Tip:

- Season with pepper and salt if needed.

Nutrition:

Calories; 280, Protein; 11.3g, Carbohydrates; 9.3g, Fat;23.5g, Cholesterol; 150.8mg, Sodium; 498.3mg.

Breakfast Socca (Farinata)

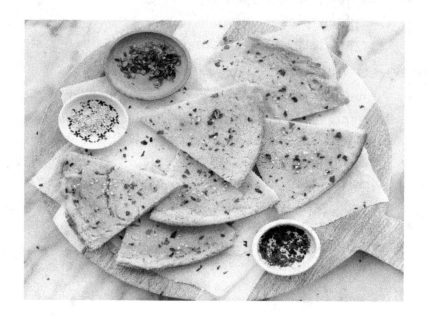

Preparation time:	Cooking time: 20 minutes	Additional time:	Servings: 4
10 minutes		2 hour	

Ingredients:

- One cup chickpea flour
- One cup water
- One tablespoon olive oil
- Half teaspoon ground cumin
- Salt and ground black pepper – to taste
- One tablespoon vegetable oil – for frying

Instructions:

- Mix water, olive oil, chickpeas, and flour into the bowl and season with pepper, salt, and cumin. Stir well until combine. Keep it aside.
- Let rest for two hours.
- Preheat the oven to 450 degrees Fahrenheit. Place the skillet into the oven and heat for five to seven minutes.
- Remove the skillet from the oven and then grease with oil, and add half of the batter into it. Place into the oven and bake for five minutes. Turn on the broiler and cook for one minute.
- Remove from the oven and repeat with the remaining batter.

Additional Tip:

- Sprinkle with parsley.

Nutrition:

Calories; 146, Protein; 4.7g, Carbohydrates; 13.8g, Fat; 8.4g, Sodium; 41mg.

Best Olive Oil and Tahini

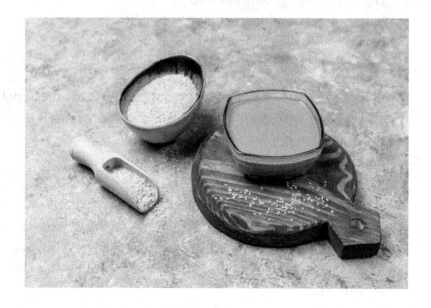

Preparation time:	Cooking time:	Servings:
15 minutes	40 minutes	14

Ingredients:

- 2 ½ cups old-fashioned rolled oats
- ¾ cup shelled pistachios
- ¾ cup walnuts
- Half cup sunflower seed
- Three tablespoons raw sesame seeds
- One cup unsweetened coconut flakes
- ¾ cup honey
- 2/3 cup tahini
- Half cup extra-virgin olive oil
- Two teaspoons pure vanilla extract
- Half cup brown sugar
- Half teaspoon ground cinnamon
- Half teaspoon cardamom
- Half cup medjool dates – about 6 dates, pitted and chopped
- Half cup dry cranberries or cherries

Instructions:

- Preheat the oven to 350 degrees Fahrenheit.
- Mix the coconut flakes, sesame seeds, sunflower seed, walnut, pistachios, and oats into the bowl.
- Combine cardamom, cinnamon, brown sugar, vanilla extract, olive oil, tahini, and honey in another bowl. Add over the oat mixture and toss to combine.
- Scatter the mixture on the sheet pan and place it into the oven and bake for seven to ten minutes until golden.
- Remove from the flame. Let cool it. Break it into clusters and combine in cranberries and dates.

Additional Tip:

- Serve with warm milk.

Nutrition

Calories; 392kcal, Carbohydrates; 40.1g, Protein; 8.1g,
Saturated Fat; 1.6g, Sodium; 11.3mg,
Potassium; 328.3mg, Fiber; 5.4g, Vitamin A; 42.8 IU,
Vitamin C; 1.2mg, Calcium; 69.7mg, Iron; 2.5mg

Delicious Raspberry Clafoutis

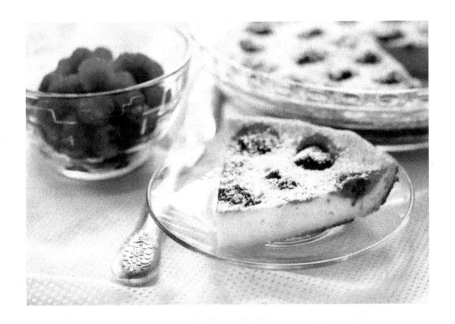

Preparation time:	Cooking time:	Servings:
15 minutes	35 minutes	6

Ingredients:

- Unsalted butter – for baking dish
- Three cups raspberries
- Half cup plus one tablespoon granulated sugar
- One teaspoon dried lavender buds
- Half cup whole milk
- Half cup crème fraiche, more – for serving
- Four eggs
- Pinch of salt
- 1/3 cup all-purpose flour
- Confectioners' sugar – for serving

Instructions:

- Preheat the oven to 375 degrees Fahrenheit. Butter the ceramic baking dish.
- Toss the raspberries with one tbsp sugar into the bowl. Let rest them.
- Mix the remaining half cup sugar and lavender into the blender. Process for two minutes. Add salt, egg, crème fraiche, and milk and mix well.
- Add the flour and again mix well.
- Place the sugared berries on the baking dish and add egg mixture over it. Place into the oven and bake for thirty-five minutes.
- Transfer the baking dish to the wire rack and cook for fifteen minutes.

Additional Tip:

- Sprinkle with confectioners' sugar.
- Serve with whipped crème fraiche.

Nutrition:

Calories; 135kcal,Carbohydrates;33.5g,Protein;5.8g,Fat;3. 9g, Saturated

Fat;1.3g,Cholesterol;111.2mg,Sodium;51.3mg,Potassium; 165.3mg,Fiber;4.1g,Vitamin A;211.1iu,Vitamin C;15.7mg,Calcium;56.2mg,Iron;1.2mg.

Tahini banana date shakes

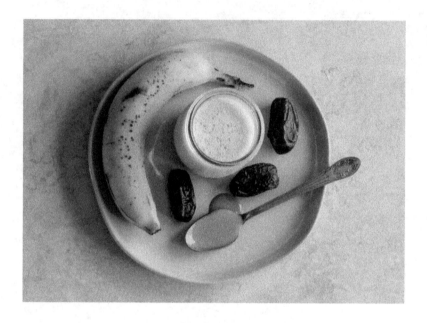

Preparation Time:	Serving:
5 minutes	2

Ingredients:

- Two frozen bananas – sliced
- Four pitted Medjool dates
- ¼ cup tahini
- ¼ cup crushed ice
- 1 ½ cups unsweetened almond milk
- Pinch ground cinnamon

Instructions:

- Add sliced frozen bananas into the blender. Add remaining ingredients and blend until creamy and smooth.
- Transfer it to the serving glass. Add ground cinnamon to it.
- Serve!

Additional Tip:

- Sprinkle with ground cinnamon.

Nutrition:

Calories; 299kcal, Total; 12.4g, Saturated Fat; 1.6g, Cholesterol; 0mg, Sodium; 102mg, Total Carb; 47.7g, Sugar; 30.9g, Protein; 5.7g

Feta and spinach frittata

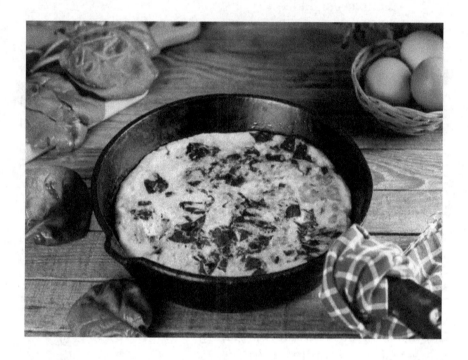

Preparation Time:	Cooking Time:	Serving:
10 minutes	12 minutes	8

Ingredients:

- Eight eggs
- ¼ cup milk
- Onetsp dried oregano
- Half tsp dill weed
- Halftsp black pepper
- Halftsp paprika
- ¼ tsp baking powder
- Pinch salt
- 6 oz frozen chopped spinach – thawed
- Half cup yellow onion – chopped
- One cup fresh parsley – chopped
- Three tbsp chopped fresh mint leaves
- Three garlic cloves – minced
- 3 to 4 oz crumbled feta cheese
- Extra virgin olive oil

Instructions:

- Preheat the oven to 375 degrees Fahrenheit.
- Whisk the pinch of salt, baking powder, spices, and egg into the bowl.
- Add spinach and remaining ingredients to the egg mixture and combine well.
- Add two tbsp olive oil into the skillet and cook until shimmering.
- Add in egg mixture. Stir well and cook for four minutes over a medium-high flame.
- Place into the oven and bake for eight minutes until cooked and firm.

Additional Tip:

- Serve with salad.

Nutrition:

Calories; 152kcal, Total Fat; 10.7g, Saturated Fat; 3.7g, Trans Fat; 0g, Sodium; 347.8mg, Total Carb; 4.9g, Sugar; 1.5g, Protein; 9.8g

Healthy Banana walnut bread

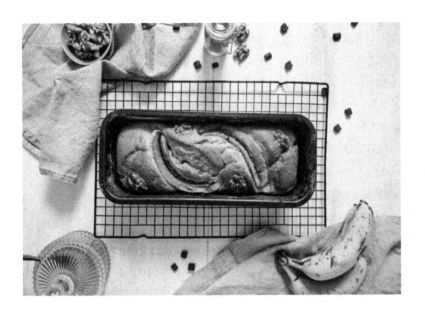

Preparation Time:	Cooking Time:	Serving:
15 minutes	55 minutes	4

Ingredients:

- 1/3 cup Greek extra virgin olive oil
- Half cup honey
- Two eggs
- Three extra ripe bananas – mashed
- Two tbsp fat free plain yogurt
- ¼ cup fat free or low-fat milk
- One tsp baking soda
- One tsp vanilla extract
- ½ to ¾ tsp ground cardamom
- Halftsp ground cinnamon
- Halftsp ground nutmeg
- 1 1/3 cup all-purpose flour
- Six dates – pitted and chopped
- 1/3 cup walnut hearts – chopped

Instructions:

- Preheat the oven to 325 degrees Fahrenheit.
- Whisk the honey and olive oil into the mixing bowl. Add the eggs and whisk well.
- Add nutmeg, cinnamon, cardamom, vanilla extract, baking soda, milk, yogurt, and banana. Whisk well.
- Add in flour, walnuts, and dates and stir the batter using a spatula and combine everything.
- Oil the loaf pan and add batter into the loaf pan. Shake well.
- Place into the oven and bake for fifty minutes at 325 degrees Fahrenheit.
- If it needs more time, bake for five minutes more.
- Remove from the oven. Let cool it for ten minutes.
- Cut and enjoy!

Additional Tip:

- Serve with jam or butter.

Nutrition:

Calories; 200kcal, total fat; 6.9g, sodium; 121.5mg, total carb; 33.6g, sugar; 22.4g, protein; 2.8g

Breakfast egg muffins

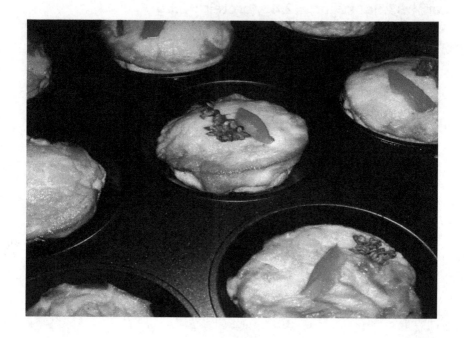

Preparation Time:	Cooking Time:	Serving:
15 minutes	25 minutes	6

Ingredients:

- Extra virgin olive oil – for brushing
- One red bell pepper – chopped
- Twelve cherry tomatoes – halved
- One shallot – chopped
- 6 to 10 pitted kalamata olives – chopped
- 3 to 4 oz cooked chicken or turkey – boneless, shredded
- 1-oz fresh parsley leaves – chopped
- Handful crumbled feta
- Eight eggs
- Salt and pepper – to taste
- Half tsp Spanish paprika
- ¼ tsp ground turmeric

Instructions:

- Preheat the oven to 350 degrees Fahrenheit.
- Prepare the twelve cups muffin pan and brush with extra-virgin olive oil.
- Split the crumbled feta, parsley, chicken or turkey, shallots, tomatoes, and peppers into the twelve cups.
- Add spices, pepper, salt, and eggs into the mixing bowl. Whisk until combine.
- Add egg mixture over each cup. Place muffin cups on top of the sheet pan. Bake for twenty-five minutes until set.
- Let cool for few minutes. Remove from the pan and serve!

Additional Tip:

- Serve with Mediterranean smoothie.

Nutrition:

Calories; 67kcal, Total fat; 4.7g, sodium; 161.4mg, total carb; 1.2g. Protein; 4.6g

Greek Salad with Edamame

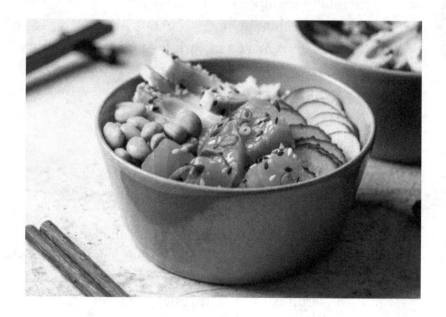

Preparation time:	Serving:
20 minutes	4

Ingredients:

- ¼ cup red-wine vinegar
- Three tablespoons extra-virgin olive oil
- ¼ teaspoon salt
- ¼ teaspoon ground pepper
- Eight cups romaine – chopped
- 16 ounces frozen shelled edamame – thawed
- One cup halved cherry or grape tomatoes
- Half European cucumber – sliced
- Half cup crumbled feta cheese
- ¼ cup slivered fresh basil
- ¼ cup Kalamata olives – sliced
- ¼ cup slivered red onion

Instructions:

- First, whisk the pepper, salt, oil, and vinegar into the bowl.
- Add onion, olives, basil, feta, cucumber, tomatoes, edamame, and romaine and toss to combine.
- Serve and enjoy!

Additional Tip:

- Sprinkle with olives and feta cheese.

Nutrition:

Calories; 344, Protein; 17.1g,Carbohydrates; 19.9g,Dietary Fiber; 8.8g,Sugars; 6.3g,Fat; 23.3g,Saturated Fat; 5.3g,Cholesterol; 16.7mg,Calcium; 216.1mg,Iron; 4.1mg,Magnesium; 101.4mg,Potassium; 907.6mg,Sodium; 488.7mg

Fig and Goat Cheese Salad

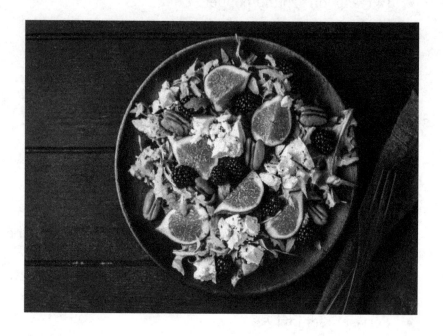

Preparation time:	Serving:
10 minutes	1

Ingredients:

- Two cups mixed salad greens
- Four dried figs – stemmed and sliced
- One-ounce fresh goat cheese – crumbled
- 1 ½ tablespoons slivered almonds – toasted
- Two teaspoons extra-virgin olive oil
- Two teaspoons balsamic vinegar
- Half teaspoon honey
- Pinch of salt
- Freshly ground pepper – to taste

Instructions:

- Mix the almonds, goat cheese, figs, and greens into the bowl.
- Add pepper, honey, salt, vinegar, and oil and combine well.
- Drizzle the dressing over the salad. Toss to combine.

Additional Tip:

- Sprinkle with sea salt and ground pepper.

Nutrition:

Calories; 340 ,Protein; 10.4g,Carbohydrates; 31.8g,Dietary Fiber; 7g,Sugars; 21.8g,Fat; 21g,Saturated Fat; 5.9g,Cholesterol; 13mg,Vitamin C; 18.1mg,Calcium; 186.1mg,Iron; 3.2mg,Magnesium; 83mg,Potassium; 676.2mg,Sodium; 309.5mg,Added Sugar ;3g.

Mediterranean Quinoa Salad

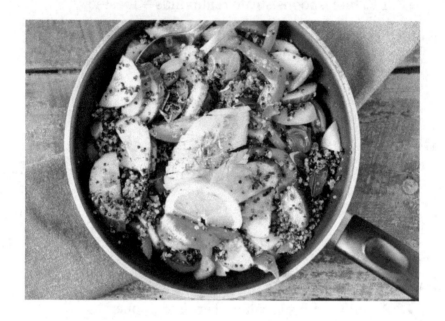

Preparation time:	**Serving**:
45 minutes	6

Ingredients:

- Half cup extra-virgin olive oil
- Six tablespoons red-wine vinegar
- Three tablespoons fresh oregano – chopped
- 1 ½ teaspoons honey
- 1 ½ teaspoons Dijon mustard
- ¼ teaspoon crushed red pepper
- Three cups cooked quinoa – cooled
- Two cups English cucumber – sliced thinly
- 1 ½ cups red onion – sliced thinly
- One cup grape tomatoes – halved
- Half cup halved pitted Kala mätä olives
- 15 ounce no-salt-added chickpeas – rinsed
- One cup crumbled feta – divided
- Three cups baby spinach

Instructions:

- Whisk the crushed red pepper, Dijon, honey, oregano, vinegar, and oil into the bowl.
- Add half cup feta, chickpeas, olives, tomatoes, onion, cucumber, and quinoa and toss to coat. Cover with lid. Place into the fridge for a half-hour.
- Add spinach and toss to coat. Sprinkle with remaining half cup feta.
- Serve!

Additional Tip:

- Add salt and lemon juice over the salad.

Nutrition:

Calories; 472, Protein; 12.1g,Carbohydrates; 39.1g,Dietary Fiber; 6.9g,Sugars; 7.4g,Fat; 30.1g,Saturated Fat; 7g,Cholesterol; 6.3mg,Calcium; 209.1mg,Iron.

Mediterranean Chicken and Broccoli Salad with Lemon Dressing

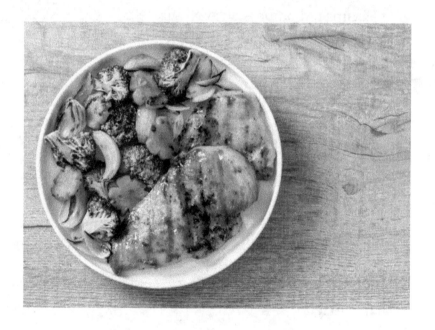

Preparation time:	Serving:
35 minutes	4

Ingredients:

- 8 ounce boneless, skinless chicken breast – trimmed
- Four tablespoons extra-virgin olive oil
- 1/8 teaspoon salt plus 1/4 teaspoon.
- Two lemons – thinly sliced and seeded
- One cup low-sodium chicken broth
- Half cup quinoa
- 8 ounces broccoli – with stems
- ¼ cup red-wine vinegar
- One tablespoon Dijon mustard
- Two cups arugula
- ¾ cup walnuts – toasted, chopped
- Half cup dried cranberries
- Half cup chopped fresh mint

Instructions:

- Preheat the oven to 425 degrees Fahrenheit.
- Add chicken to the rimmed baking sheet.
- Drizzle with one tbsp oil. Sprinkle with 1/8 tsp salt.
- Cook for ten minutes. Place lemon slices on the baking sheet.
- Cook for seven to nine minutes.
- During this, add quinoa and broth into the saucepan. Decrease the speed of the flame and cover with a lid. Cook for fifteen minutes.
- Remove from the flame. Let rest for ten minutes.
- Slice broccoli florets from the stems. Trim and peel and cut the stems and then chop the florets into pieces.
- Next, chop half of the lemon slices. Mix in the big bowl with ¼ tsp salt, three tbsp oil, mustard, and vinegar.
- Cut the chicken. Add mint, cranberries, walnuts, arugula, quinoa, broccoli, chicken and remaining lemon slices to the dressing and toss to coat. Serve!

Additional Tip:

- Sprinkle with crumbled bacon.

Nutrition:

Calories; 481, Protein; 21.5g,Carbohydrates; 43g,Dietary Fiber; 7.9g,Sugars; 18.8g,Fat; 26.5g,Saturated Fat; 3.2g,Cholesterol; 31.3mg,Calcium; 140mg,Iron; 3.2mg,Magnesium; 83.1mg,Potassium; 584.5mg,Sodium; 365.5mg,Added Sugar; 12g.

Healthy Tomato, Cucumber & White-Bean Salad

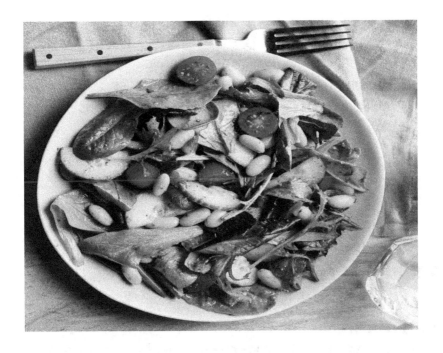

Preparation time:	Serving:
25 minutes	4

Ingredients:

- Half cup fresh basil leaves
- ¼ cup extra-virgin olive oil
- Three tablespoons red-wine vinegar
- One tablespoon shallot – chopped
- Two teaspoons Dijon mustard
- One teaspoon honey
- ¼ teaspoon salt
- ¼ teaspoon ground pepper
- 10 cups mixed salad greens
- 15 ounce low-sodium cannellini beans – rinsed
- One cup halved cherry or grape tomatoes
- Half cucumber – halved lengthwise and sliced

Instructions:

- Add pepper, salt, honey, mustard, shallot, vinegar, oil, and basil into the food processor.
- Process until smooth.
- Transfer to the bowl. Add cucumber, tomatoes, and greens, and beans and toss to combine.

Additional Tip:

- Top with fresh herbs.

Nutrition:

Calories; 246, Protein; 7.5g,Carbohydrates; 21.5g,Dietary Fiber; 7.6g,Sugars; 4.9g,Fat; 15.3g,Saturated Fat; 2g,Vitamin A; I 4400.6IU, Vitamin C; 29.9mg,Calcium; 125.6mg,Iron; 3.6mg,Magnesium; 90.7mg,Potassium; 793.3mg,Sodium; 270.5mg,Added Sugar; 1g.

Mediterranean Broccoli Pasta Salad

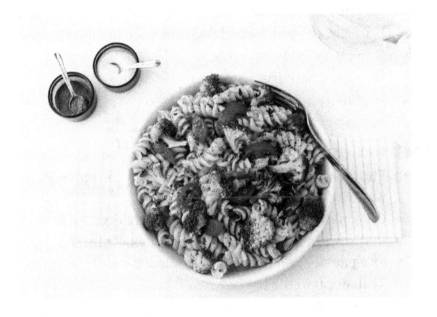

Preparation time:	Serving:
25 minutes	10

Ingredients:

- Eight ounces whole-wheat farfalle pasta
- Six cups broccoli florets
- Half cup red bell pepper – chopped
- ¼ cup red onion – chopped
- Two tablespoons fresh flat-leaf parsley – chopped
- Two tablespoons fresh basil – chopped
- ¾ cup mayonnaise
- Half cup chopped sun-dried tomatoes in oil – drained
- One teaspoon lemon zest
- One teaspoon dried oregano
- Half teaspoon salt
- ¼ teaspoon crushed red pepper

Instructions:

- First, place a big bowl of ice water near the stove. Boil the water.
- Cook pasta according to packet instruction. Add broccoli to the water and cook for two minutes. Drain the broccoli and pasta. Then, transfer it to the ice water. Drain it.
- Transfer it to the big bowl. Add basil, parsley, onion, and bell pepper.
- Mix the crushed red pepper, salt, oregano, lemon zest, sun-dried tomatoes, and mayonnaise into the bowl. After that, add to the pasta mixture. Toss to combine. Serve!

Additional Tip:

- Add crushed red pepper if required.

Nutrition:

Calories; 222, Protein;5.2g,Carbohydrates; 21.9g,Dietary Fiber; 3.6g; Sugars; 1.4g,Fat; 13.7g,Saturated Fat; 2.1g,Cholesterol; 7mg,Vitamin C; 56.8mg,Calcium; 39.8mg,Iron; 1.5mg,Magnesium; 50.5mg,Potassium; 312.2mg,Sodium; 250.5mg,Thiamin; 0.2mg.

Chicken &Faro Herb Salad

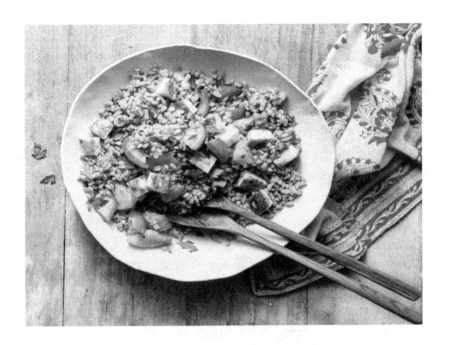

Preparation time:	Serving:
1 hour	6

Ingredients:

Red-Wine Vinaigrette:
- 1/3 cup red-wine vinegar
- 1 ½ tbsp Dijon mustard
- One clove garlic – minced
- ¾ teaspoon kosher salt
- Half teaspoon ground pepper
- Half cup extra-virgin olive oil

Salad:
- Three cups water
- One cup farro
- 1 ½ pounds boneless, skinless chicken breast – trimmed
- Half teaspoon kosher salt
- ¼ teaspoon ground pepper
- One fennel bulb – cored and chopped
- One cup carrot – diced
- One cup English cucumber – chopped, seeded
- Half cup red onion – chopped
- ¼ cup flat-leaf parsley – chopped
- ¼ cup fresh basil, very thinly sliced
- ¼ cup fresh mint – very thinly sliced
- Two cups arugula – tough stems removed, coarsely chopped
- ¼ cup oil-cured black olives – sliced

Instructions:

- **Prepare the vinaigrette:** First, whisk the half tsp pepper, ¾ tsp salt, garlic, mustard, and vinegar into the bowl. Whisk in the oil.
- **Prepare the salad:** Add water into the saucepan and boil it. Add farro and then decrease the speed of the flame to low. Let simmer for fifteen to twenty-five

minutes. Drain it. Then, transfer the farro to the big bowl.

- After that, toss 1/3 cup of vinaigrette with hot farro. Let rest until cool.
- Preheat the grill to medium-high flame.
- Next, sprinkle the chicken with pepper and salt. Grill chicken for twelve to sixteen minutes. Let rest for five minutes. Cut it.
- Add 1/3 vinaigrette, mint, basil, parsley, onion, cucumber, carrot, and fennel into the farro.
- Add arugula into the farro mixture. Top with olives and chicken.
- Drizzle with vinaigrette.

Additional Tip:
- Garnish with cilantro.

Nutrition:
Calories; 459, Protein; 28.2g,Carbohydrates; 31.9g,Dietary Fiber; 5.3g,Sugars; 4.8g,Fat; 24.5g,Saturated Fat; 3.7g,Cholesterol; 62.7mg,Vitamin A; Iu 4562.4IU,Vitamin C; 12.7mg,Calcium; 86.4mg,Iron; 2.7mg,Sodium; 512.6mg

Green Salad with Pita Bread & Hummus

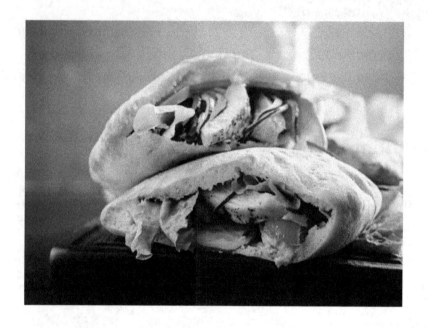

Preparation time:	Serving:
10 minutes	1

Ingredients:

- Two cups mixed salad greens
- Half cup cucumber – sliced
- Two tablespoons grated carrot
- 1 ½ teaspoons extra-virgin olive oil
- 1 ½ teaspoons balsamic vinegar
- Pinch of salt
- Pinch of ground pepper
- One whole-wheat pita bread – toasted, 6 ½-inch
- ¼ cup hummus

Instructions:

- Place carrot, cucumber, and greens on the plate.
- Drizzle with vinegar and oil.
- Sprinkle with pepper and salt.

Additional Tip:

- Serve with hummus and pita.

Nutrition:

Calories; 374, Protein; 13.5g,Carbohydrates; 52.6g,Dietary Fiber; 10.7g,Sugars; 5.3g,Fat; 14.5g,Saturated Fat; 2g,Vitamin C; 20mg,Calcium; 109.4mg,Iron; 5.2mg,Magnesium; 124.6mg,Potassium; 732.1mg,Sodium; 759.8mg

White Bean & Veggie Salad

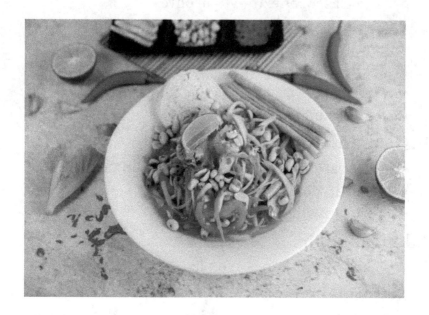

Preparation time:	**Serving**:
10 minutes	1

Ingredients:

- Two cups mixed salad greens
- ¾ cup veggies – cucumbers and cherry tomatoes
- 1/3 cup white beans – rinsed and drained
- Half avocado – diced
- One tablespoon red-wine vinegar
- Two teaspoons extra-virgin olive oil
- ¼ teaspoon kosher salt
- Freshly ground pepper – to taste

Instructions:

- Mix the avocado, beans, veggies, and greens into the bowl.
- Drizzle with oil and vinegar – season with pepper and salt.
- Toss to coat and then add to the big plate.

Additional Tip:

- Sprinkle with fresh herbs.

Nutrition:

Calories; 360, Protein; 10.1g,Carbohydrates; 29.7g,Dietary Fiber; 13.3g,Sugars; 2.9g, Fat; 24.6g,Saturated Fat; 3.6g,Vitamin C; 30mg,Calcium; 140.1mg,Iron; 4.5mg,Magnesium; 104mg,Potassium; 1291.6mg,Sodium; 321.3mg

Watermelon, Olive, Caper & Feta Salad

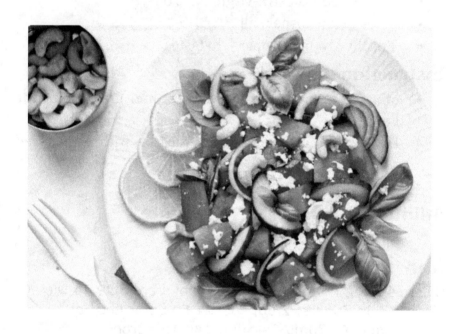

Preparation time:	Serving:
30 minutes	6

Ingredients:

- Two tablespoons extra-virgin olive oil – plus 1/4 cup
- ¼ cup rinsed capers
- 1/3 cup pitted Kalamata olives – halved
- 1 ½ tablespoons sherry vinegar
- Ground pepper – to taste
- Five cups watermelon – diced
- Half cup fresh basil – thinly sliced
- Half cup fresh mint – thinly sliced
- 2/3 cup crumbled feta cheese
- ¼ cup sliced almonds – toasted
- Flaky sea salt – for garnish

Instructions:

- Add two tbsp oil into a saucepan and cook over a high flame.
- Add capers dry and then add to the hot oil. Cook for one to three minutes until crisp. Transfer it to the plate using a spoon.
- Next, whisk ¼ cup oil into the bowl with ground pepper, vinegar, and olives. Add mint, basil, and watermelon and toss to combine.
- Add into the serving bowl.

Additional Tip:

- Sprinkle with capers, almonds, and feta.
- Garnish with sea salt.

Nutrition:

Calories; 260, Protein;4.4g,Carbohydrates; 12.7g,Dietary Fiber; 1.8g,Sugars; 8.7g,Fat; 22.1g,Saturated Fat; 4.7g,Cholesterol; 14.8mg,Vitamin A; Iu 1293.8IU,Vitamin C; 12.1mg,Calcium; 125.2mg,Iron; 1.7mg,Magnesium; 35.2mg,Potassium; 228.5mg,Sodium; 356mg.

Farro, Kale & Squash Salad

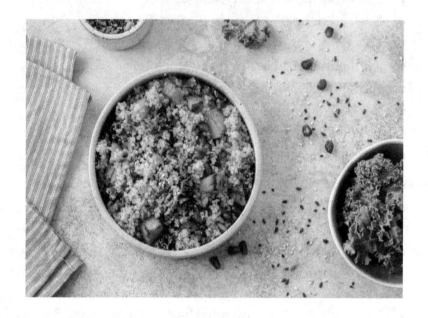

Preparation time:	Serving:
1 hour	6

Ingredients:

Farro:
- ¾ cup farro
- 1 ½ cups water
- Pinch of salt

Squash:
- Four cups cubed butternut squash
- One tablespoon extra-virgin olive oil
- ¼ teaspoon salt
- ¼ teaspoon ground pepper

Kale:
- Seven tablespoons extra-virgin olive oil
- Five tablespoons red-wine vinegar
- Three cloves garlic – minced
- Two tablespoons minced shallot
- One tablespoon Dijon mustard
- ¼ teaspoon salt plus 1/8 teaspoon
- ¼ teaspoon ground pepper plus 1/8 teaspoon
- One bunch kale
- 1 ¼ cups water
- Half cup crumbled feta cheese
- ¼ cup toasted pepitas

Instructions:

- Preheat the oven to 425 degrees Fahrenheit. Coat the rimmed baking sheet with cooking spray.
- Prepare farro: First, toast farro into the saucepan over a medium flame until fragrant for two minutes.
- Add a pinch of salt and 1 ½ cup water and boil it.
- Decrease the speed of the flame. Let simmer it. Cover with lid.
- Cook for twenty-five to thirty-five minutes. Drain it.

- **Prepare squash:** Toss squash with pepper, salt, and one tbsp oil.
- Scatter on the baking sheet and cook for twenty to twenty-five minutes.
- **Prepare kale:** Mix the pepper, salt, mustard, shallot, garlic, vinegar, and six tbsp oil into the bowl. Split kale leaves from the stem.
- Cut the leaves crosswise into the strips and then add them to the bowl.
- Rub the dressing into the leaves.
- Add the remaining one tbsp oil into the skillet and cook over a medium-high flame.
- Add kale stems and remaining salt and pepper and cook for one to two minutes.
- Add ¼ cup water and cover with lid. Cook for two minutes.
- Transfer to the cutting board. Cut into two-inch pieces.
- Assemble: Add squash and farro into the kale salad and place on the serving plate.

Additional Tip:
- Top with pepitas, feta, and kale stems.

Nutrition:
Calories; 372, Protein; 8.4g,Carbohydrates; 30.6g,Dietary Fiber; 5.9g,Sugars; 3.9g,Fat; 25.3g,Saturated Fat; 5g,Cholesterol; 11.1mg,Vitamin A; Iu 11663.2IU,Vitamin C; 45.5mg,Calcium; 156.4mg,Magnesium; 73.1mg,Potassium; 436.5mg,Sodium; 449.9mg.

White Bean Salad with Swordfish

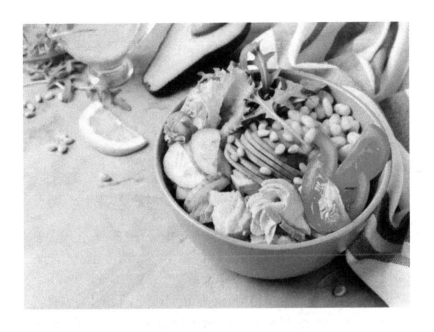

Preparation time:	Serving:
30 minutes	4

Ingredients:

- ¼ cup extra-virgin olive oil
- Two tablespoons lemon juice
- One teaspoon Dijon mustard
- Half teaspoon salt
- Half teaspoon ground pepper
- 15-ounce white beans – rinsed
- 10-ounce swordfish steaks
- One teaspoon herbs de Provence
- 12 cups escarole – chopped
- ¼ cup red onion – very thinly sliced

Instructions:

- Preheat the broiler over high. Line a broiler-safe pan with foil.
- Next, whisk the pepper, salt, mustard, lemon juice, and oil into the bowl. Transfer two tbsp of the dressing to the bowl.
- Add beans to the dressing into the big bowl.
- Toss to coat. Slice each swordfish steak in half. Sprinkle with pepper and salt and herbs de Provence.
- Place on the pan and broil for eight to ten minutes.
- Toss onion and escarole with the beans.

Additional Tip:

- Serve with swordfish and drizzle with two tbsp dressing.

Nutrition:

Calories; 397, Protein; 31.5g,Carbohydrates; 20.7gk,Dietary Fiber; 9.4g,Sugars; 1.6g,Fat; 23g,Saturated Fat; 4g,Cholesterol; 80.7mg,Vitamin A; Iu 3386.2IU,Vitamin C; 13.2mg,Calcium; 132.8mg,Iron; 2.8mg,Magnesium; 60.4mg,Potassium; 1272.1mg,Sodium; 664mg

Mediterranean Cucumber Salad

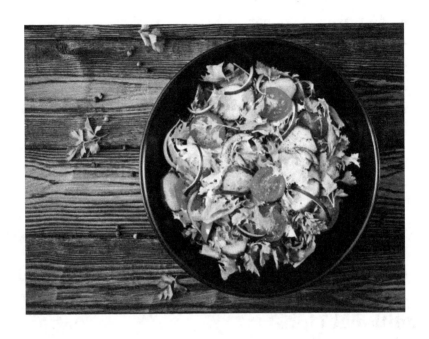

Preparation time:	Serving:
20 minutes	6

Ingredients:

- ¼ cup extra-virgin olive oil
- Two tablespoons red-wine vinegar
- One tablespoon fresh oregano – for garnish, chopped
- ¼ teaspoon salt
- ¼ teaspoon pepper
- One cucumber
- One cup cherry tomatoes – halved
- Half cup red onion – thinly sliced
- Half cup cubed feta cheese
- ¼ cup Kalamata olives – sliced, pitted

Instructions:

- Whisk the pepper, salt, oregano, vinegar, and oil into the bowl.
- Cut the cucumber into noodles using a vegetable slicer. Slice the noodles into two-inch lengths.
- Add olives, cheese, onion, tomatoes, and cucumber noodles into the bowl. Toss to combine with dressing.

Additional Tip:

- Top with oregano. Serve!

Nutrition:

Calories; 149, Protein; 2.6g,Carbohydrates; 4.9g,Dietary Fiber; 0.8g,Sugars; 2.5g,Fat; 13.4g,Saturated Fat; 3.4g,Cholesterol; 11.1mg,Vitamin A; Iu 358.6IU,Vitamin C; 6.5mg,Calcium; 80.2mg,Iron; 0.4mg,Magnesium; 13.9mg,Potassium; 169.2mg,Sodium; 291.8mg.

Greek Hummus Salad

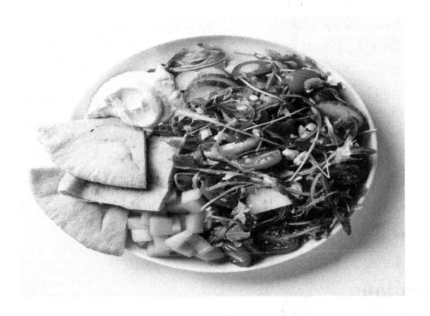

Preparation time:	Serving:
10 minutes	1

Ingredients:

- Two cups arugula
- 1/3 cup cherry tomatoes – halved
- 1/3 cup sliced cucumber
- One tablespoon red onion – chopped
- 1 ½ tablespoons extra-virgin olive oil
- Two teaspoons red-wine vinegar
- ⅛ teaspoon ground pepper
- One tablespoon feta cheese
- One whole-wheat pita – 4-inch
- ¼ cup hummus

Instructions:

- Toss arugula into the bowl with pepper, vinegar, oil, onion, cucumber, and tomatoes. Top with feta cheese.

Additional Tip:

- Serve with hummus and pita.

Nutrition:

Calories;422 ,Protein; 10.9g,Carbohydrates; 30.5g,Dietary Fiber; 7.3g,Sugars; 4.3g,Fat; 29.9g,Saturated Fat; 5.3g,Cholesterol; 8.3mg,Vitamin A; Iu 1456.6iu,Vitamin C; 15mg,Calcium; 153.5mg,Iron; 3.3mg,Magnesium; 96.9mg,Potassium; 543.8mg,Sodium; 485.8mg.

Mediterranean Lentil & Kale Salad

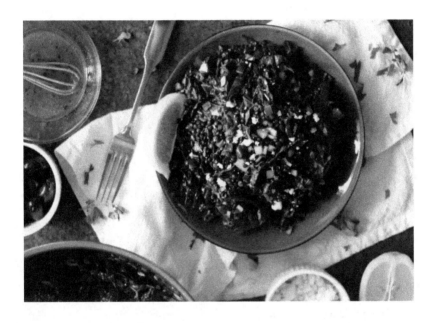

Preparation time:	Serving:
15 minutes	4

Ingredients:

- ¼ cup red wine vinegar
- Two tablespoons olive oil
- One tablespoon dried tomatoes – chopped
- One clove garlic – minced
- Half teaspoon Dijon-style mustard
- ¼ teaspoon salt
- ¼ teaspoon black pepper
- 5-ounce fresh baby kale
- 9-ounce lentils – refrigerated, steamed
- One cup red sweet pepper – chopped
- ¼ cup shredded Parmesan cheese

Instructions:

- For vinaigrette: Whisk the pepper, salt, mustard, garlic, chopped dried tomatoes, olive oil, and red wine vinegar into serving bowl.
- Add the kale and toss to combine.
- Top with sweet pepper and lentils.

Additional Tip:

- Sprinkle with cheese.

Nutrition:

Calories; 186, Protein; 9.6g,Carbohydrates; 18.2g,Dietary Fiber; 7.4g,Sugars; 3.2g,Fat; 8.6g,Saturated Fat; 1.8g,Cholesterol; 3.6mg,Vitamin C; 49mg,Calcium; 215.8mg,Iron; 3.6mg,Magnesium; 10.4mg,Potassium; 376.2mg,Sodium; 464.1mg.

Quinoa Chickpea Salad with Roasted Red Pepper

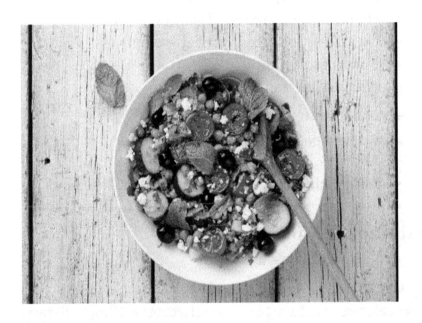

Preparation time:	Serving:
10 minutes	1

Ingredients:

- Two tablespoons hummus – roasted red pepper flavor
- One tablespoon lemon juice
- One tablespoon roasted red pepper – chopped
- Two cups mixed salad greens
- Half cup cooked quinoa
- Half cup chickpeas – rinsed
- One tablespoon unsalted sunflower seeds
- One tablespoon fresh parsley – chopped
- Pinch of salt
- Pinch of ground pepper

Instructions:

- Add red pepper, lemon juice, and hummus into the dish. Add water to thin it for dressing.
- Add chickpeas, quinoa, and greens into the bowl.
- Top with pepper, salt, parsley, and sunflower seeds.

Additional Tip:

- Serve with dressing.

Nutrition:

379 calories; protein 16g; carbohydrates 58.5g; dietary fiber 13.2g; sugars 2.9g; fat 10.5g; saturated fat 1.3g; vitamin a iu 4185.4IU; vitamin c 45.3mg; calcium 138.7mg; iron 5.8mg; magnesium 155.9mg; potassium 891.7mg; sodium 606.8mg;

Pita Panzanella Salad with Meatballs

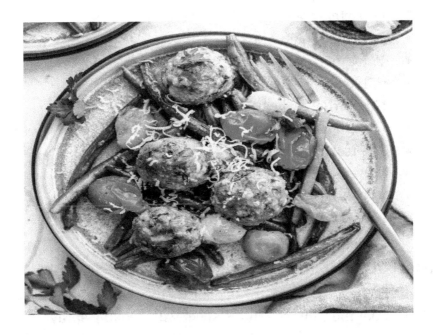

Preparation time:	Serving:
50 minutes	6

Ingredients:

- 1 ½ pounds 93%-lean ground turkey
- Half cup panko breadcrumbs
- ¼ cup grated red onion – plus 3/4 cup quartered and thinly sliced
- One egg – beaten
- One tablespoon minced fresh oregano
- Three teaspoons garlic – minced
- Two teaspoons olive oil
- ¾ teaspoon salt
- Half teaspoon ground pepper
- Three whole-wheat pita breads – six-inch
- Three tablespoons red-wine vinegar
- One teaspoon honey
- One teaspoon Dijon mustard
- One English cucumber – sliced
- 1 ¾ cups plum tomato – diced
- ¾ cup Kalamata olives – sliced, pitted

Instructions:

- Preheat the oven to 425 degrees Fahrenheit.
- Coat the rimmed baking sheet with cooking spray.
- Combine pepper, salt, two tsp oil, two tsp garlic, one tbsp oregano, egg, grated onion, breadcrumbs, and turkey into the bowl.
- Make forty-two meatballs from the mixture and place them on the baking sheet. Place into the oven and bake for ten to twelve minutes.
- Divide pita in half into thin rounds and then rear into a half-moon shape. Place on the baking sheet and bake for five to seven minutes.

- Let cool it. Break into bite-sized pieces. Whisk mustard, honey, one tsp garlic, two tsp oregano, and three tbsp oil into the bowl.
- Add sliced onion, olives, cucumber, and tomatoes and add in a pita.
- Serve with meatballs.

Additional Tip:
- Garnish with fresh herbs.

Nutrition:
380 calories; protein 34g; carbohydrates 30g; dietary fiber 4g; sugars 5g; fat 15g; saturated fat 4g; cholesterol 76mg; potassium 290mg; sodium 698mg.

Greens Pesto Chicken Salad

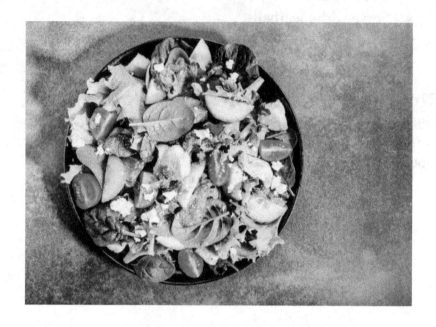

Preparation time:	**Serving**:
30 minutes	4

Ingredients:

- One pound boneless, skinless chicken breast – trimmed
- ¼ cup pesto
- ¼ cup low-fat mayonnaise
- Three tablespoons red onion – chopped
- Two tablespoons extra-virgin olive oil
- Two tablespoons red-wine vinegar
- ¼ teaspoon salt
- ¼ teaspoon ground pepper
- 5-ounce mixed salad greens
- One pint grape or cherry tomatoes – halved

Instructions:

- Add chicken into the saucepan, and then add water. Boil it.
- Cover with lid. Decrease the speed of the flame to low. Let simmer for ten to fifteen minutes.
- Transfer to the cutting board and cut into bite-sized pieces. Let cool it.
- Mix the onion, mayonnaise, and pesto into the bowl. Add chicken and toss to combine.
- Whisk the pepper, salt, oil, and vinegar into the bowl.
- Add tomatoes and greens and toss to combine.
- Split the green salad between four plates.
- Top with chicken salad.

Additional Tip:

- Top with basil leaves.

Nutrition:

324 calories; protein 27.1g; carbohydrates 9.2g; dietary fiber 2.3g; sugars 3.2g; fat 19.7g; saturated fat 4.1g; cholesterol 71.4mg; vitamin c 17.6mg; calcium 153mg.

Warm Fava Bean & Escarole Salad

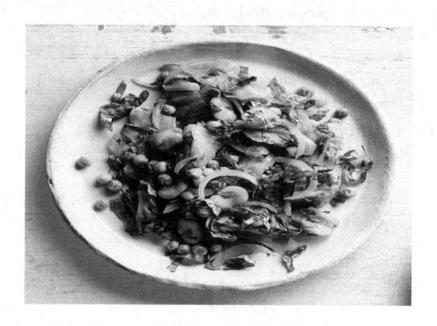

Preparation time:	Serving:
15 minutes	4

Ingredients:

- Two tablespoons extra-virgin olive oil
- One onion – halved and sliced
- Two cloves garlic – minced
- ⅛ teaspoon crushed red pepper
- Four cups escarole – chopped
- One cup shelled fresh fava beans
- One cup peas – fresh or frozen
- Half teaspoon salt
- ¼ teaspoon ground pepper
- ¼ cup fresh basil and/or mint – chopped

Instructions:

- Add oil into a saucepan and cook over a medium flame.
- Add crushed red pepper, garlic, and onion and cook for two to three minutes.
- Add pepper, salt, peas, beans, and escarole and cook for two to three minutes. Remove from the flame.

Additional Tip:

- Top with fresh herbs.

Nutrition:

237 calories; protein 12.6g; carbohydrates 30.7g; dietary fiber 12.8g; sugars 5.1g; fat 7.8g; saturated fat 1.1g; vitamin c 19.8mg; folate 240.7mcg; calcium 79.5mg; iron 3.5mg; magnesium 93.8mg; potassium 646.9mg; sodium 306.7mg

Tomato & Onion Salad with Tofu

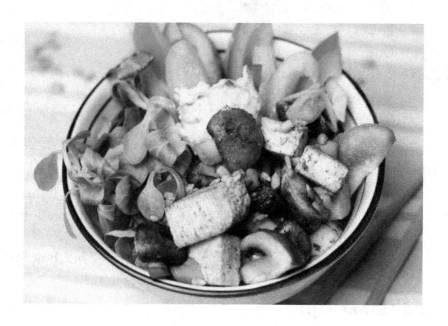

Preparation time:	Serving:
3 hours 45 minutes	4

Ingredients:

Crispy Tofu:
- 14- to-16-ounce extra-firm water-packed tofu – drained
- Five tablespoons extra-virgin olive oil
- ¼ cup lemon juice
- Two tablespoons fresh basil – chopped
- Two teaspoons fresh oregano – chopped
- One teaspoon ground pepper
- 1/8 teaspoon kosher salt
- ¼ cup all-purpose flour
- Two eggs
- 2/3 cup grated Parmesan cheese
- 1/3 cup whole-wheat panko breadcrumbs

Salad:
- Four ripe tomatoes – each cut into six wedges
- Two cups sweet onion – thinly sliced, halved
- Half cup Castelvetrano olives
- ¼ cup Kalamata olives – chopped, pitted
- Three tablespoons fresh basil – chopped
- Two teaspoons fresh oregano – chopped
- Three tablespoons extra-virgin olive oil
- Two tablespoons red-wine vinegar
- One tablespoon lemon juice
- ¼ teaspoon ground pepper
- 1/8 teaspoon kosher salt

Instructions:

- **Marinate the tofu:** Slice tofu crosswise into eight pieces. Press or one to four hours.
- Mix the 1/8 tsp salt, one tsp pepper, two tsp oregano, two tbsp basil, ¼ cup lemon juice, and two tbsp oil on the baking dish.

- Add pressed tofu and coat well. Cover with lid. Place into the fridge for two hours.
- **Prepare the salad:** Toss the salt, pepper, lemon juice, vinegar, oil, one tsp oregano, two tbsp basil, olives, onion, and tomatoes into the bowl. Keep it aside.
- Cook the tofu: Remove the marinade and pat dry tofu. Add flour into the dish. Beat eggs in another dish. Mix the panko and parmesan cheese in another bowl. Immerse the tofu in the flour and shake well. Then, dip in egg and then immerse in cheese mixture. Press it.
- Add two tbsp oil into the skillet and cook over a medium-high flame. Add half of the tofu and cook over a medium flame for two to four minutes. Place on the paper towel.
- Transfer the salad to the serving bowl.

Additional Tip:

- Top with one tsp oregano, one tbsp basil, and tofu.

Nutrition:

549 calories; protein 17.6g; carbohydrates 23g; dietary fiber 5.1g; sugars 6.8g; fat 43.8g; saturated fat 6.6g; cholesterol 55.1mg; vitamin c 28.4mg; calcium 441.5mg; iron 3.9mg; magnesium 65.2mg; potassium 586.8mg; sodium 641.4mg.

Roasted Salmon and Chickpeas & Greens

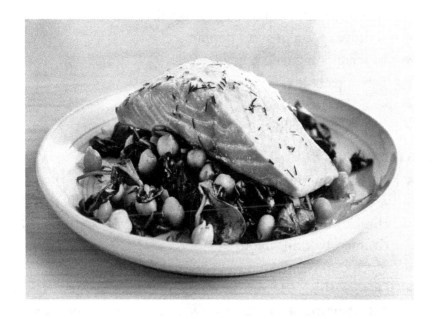

Preparation time:	Serving:
40 minutes	4

Ingredients:

- Two tablespoons extra-virgin olive oil
- One tablespoon smoked paprika
- Half teaspoon salt
- 15 ounce no-salt-added chickpeas – rinsed
- 1/3 cup buttermilk
- ¼ cup mayonnaise
- ¼ cup chopped fresh chives or dill – for garnish
- Half teaspoon ground pepper
- ¼ teaspoon garlic powder
- Ten cups kale – chopped
- ¼ cup water
- 1 ¼ pounds wild salmon – cut into 4 portions

Instruction:

- Preheat the oven to 425 degrees Fahrenheit.
- Add ¼ tsp salt, paprika, and one tbsp oil into a bowl. Pat chicken dry. Toss with paprika mixture. Scatter on the rimmed baking sheet.
- Place into the oven and bake for a half-hour.
- During this, add garlic powder, ¼ tsp pepper, herbs, mayonnaise, and buttermilk into the blender. Keep it aside.
- Add one tbsp oil into the skillet and cook over a medium flame. Add kale and cook for two minutes. Add water and cook for five minutes until tender.
- Remove from the flame and add salt. Remove the chickpeas from the oven and then add to the pan. Add salmon and season with pepper and salt. Place into the oven and bake for five to eight minutes.
- Drizzle the reserved dressing over the salmon.

Additional Tip:

- Garnish with herbs. Serve with chickpeas and kale.

Nutrition:

447 calories; protein 37g; carbohydrates 23.4g; dietary
fiber 6.4g; sugars 2.2g; fat 21.8g; saturated fat 3.7g;
cholesterol 72.9mg; vitamin c 51.7mg; calcium 197.8mg;
iron 3mg; magnesium 99.4mg; potassium 990.8mg;
sodium 556.7mg.

Mediterranean Cod with Roasted Tomatoes

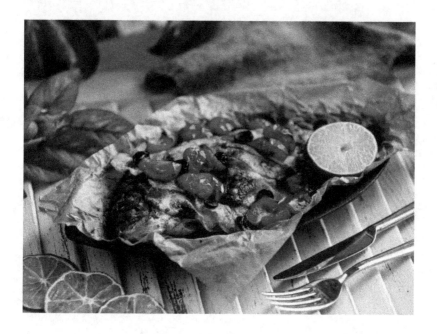

Preparation time:	Serving:
15 minutes	4

Ingredients:

- Four fresh or frozen skinless cod fillets – 3/4- to 1- inches thick, four-ounce
- Two teaspoons fresh oregano – snipped
- One teaspoon fresh thyme – snipped
- Half teaspoon salt
- ¼ teaspoon garlic powder
- ¼ teaspoon paprika
- ¼ teaspoon black pepper
- Nonstick cooking spray
- Three cups cherry tomatoes
- Two cloves garlic – sliced
- One tablespoon olive oil
- Two tablespoons ripe olives – pitted, sliced
- Two teaspoons capers
- Fresh oregano or thyme leaves

Instruction:

- Preheat the oven to 450 degrees Fahrenheit. Wash fish and pat dry with a paper towel. Mix the black pepper, paprika, garlic powder, salt, snipped thyme and snipped oregano into the bowl.
- Sprinkle with half of the oregano mixture. Line the baking pan with foil.
- Coat foil with cooking spray. Add fish to the foiled pan. Add garlic and tomatoes on the other side of the foiled pan.
- Mix the remaining oregano mixture with oil. Drizzle oil mixture over the tomatoes and toss to combine. Place into the oven and bake for eight to twelve minutes. Add capers and olives into the cooked tomato mixture.
- Split roasted tomato mixture and fish between four serving plates.

Additional Tip:

- Garnish with thyme leaves or oregano.

Nutrition:

157 calories; protein 21.6g; carbohydrates 6.5g; dietary fiber 1.8g; sugars 3.6g; fat 4.8g; saturated fat 0.8g; cholesterol 48.8mg; vitamin a iu 1267.7IU; vitamin c 21.1mg; calcium 40.6mg; iron 1mg; magnesium 53.5mg; potassium 807mg; sodium 429.2mg.

Linguine with Creamy White Clam Sauce

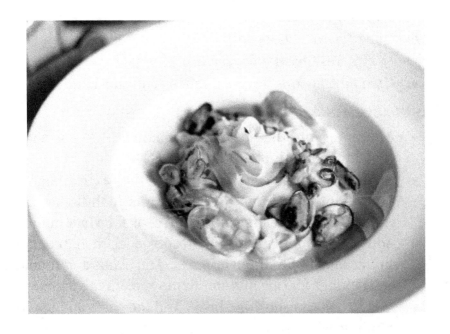

Preparation time:	Serving:
15 minutes	4

Ingredients:

- 8-ounces whole-wheat linguine
- 16-ounce clams – chopped
- Three tablespoons extra-virgin olive oil
- Three cloves garlic – chopped
- ¼ teaspoon crushed red pepper
- One tablespoon lemon juice
- ¼ teaspoon salt
- One tomato – chopped
- ¼ cup fresh basil – for garnish, chopped
- Two tablespoons heavy cream or half-and-half

Instructions:

- Add water into the saucepan and boil it. Add pasta and cook for eight minutes until tender. Drain it.
- During this, drain clams and reserve the ¾ cup of liquid. Add oil into the skillet over a medium-high flame. Add crushed red pepper and garlic and cook for a half minute. Add salt, lemon juice, and reserved clam liquid. Let simmer for two to three minutes. Add clams and tomato and simmer for one minute. Remove from the flame.
- Add in half-and-half and basil. Add the pasta and toss to combine with sauce.

Additional Tip:

- Garnish with basil.

Nutrition:

421 calories; protein 21.5g; carbohydrates 51.9g; dietary fiber 7.8g; sugars 3.8g; fat 16.6g; saturated fat 3.6g; cholesterol 48.2mg; vitamin a iu 682.5IU; vitamin c 10.4mg; calcium 61.5mg; iron 5mg; magnesium 91.8mg; potassium 286.6mg; sodium 371.9mg; thiamin 0.3mg.

Yummy Shrimp Scampi

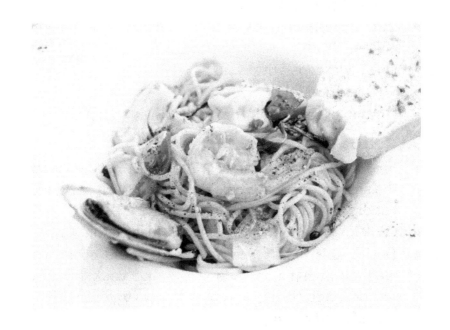

Preparation time:	**Serving**:
20 minutes	4

Ingredients:

- 1 ½ pounds fresh or frozen shrimp in shells
- 6-ounces whole-wheat or plain linguine
- One tablespoon olive oil
- Three cloves garlic – minced
- Two tablespoons dry white wine or reduced-sodium chicken broth
- One tablespoon butter
- 1/8 teaspoon salt
- One tablespoon fresh chives or parsley – chopped

Instructions:

- First, thaw shrimp if frozen. After that, devein and peel the shrimp and leave tails if desired. Wash shrimp and pat dry with a paper towel.
- Cook linguine according to packet instruction. Drain it.
- During this, add oil into the skillet and cook over a medium-high flame. Add garlic and cook for fifteen seconds. Add shrimp and cook for two to four minutes.
- Transfer the shrimp to the serving plate.
- Add salt, butter, and wine to the skillet and cook over a medium flame. Add butter mixture over the shrimp.

Additional Tip:

- Sprinkle with chives. Serve over linguine.

Nutrition:

341 calories; protein 29g; carbohydrates 34g; dietary fiber 1g; sugars 2g; fat 9g; saturated fat 3g; cholesterol 222mg; vitamin a iu 476IU; vitamin c 2mg; calcium 107mg; iron 2mg; magnesium 62mg; potassium 274mg; sodium 1039mg.

Salmon with Roasted Red Pepper Quinoa Salad

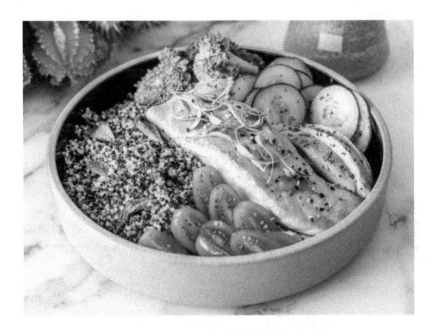

Preparation time:	Serving:
15 minutes	4

Ingredients:

- Three tablespoons extra-virgin olive oil
- 1 ¼ pounds skin-on salmon – cut into 4 portions
- Half teaspoon salt
- Half teaspoon ground pepper
- Two tablespoons red-wine vinegar
- One clove garlic – grated
- Two cups cooked quinoa
- One cup roasted red bell peppers – rinsed, chopped
- ¼ cup fresh cilantro – chopped
- ¼ cup chopped toasted pistachios

Instructions:

- Add one tbsp oil into the skillet and cook over a medium flame.
- Pat salmon dry with a paper towel and sprinkle with pepper and salt.
- Add it to the pan and cook for three to four minutes. Turnover and cook for one to two minutes. Transfer it to the big plate.
- During this, whisk garlic, vinegar, pepper, salt, and two tbsp oil into the bowl. Add pistachios, cilantro, pepper, and quinoa and toss to coat.

Additional Tip:

- Serve with salad.

Nutrition:

481 calories; protein 35.8g; carbohydrates 31g; dietary fiber 3.5g; sugars 1.4g; fat 21g; saturated fat 3.4g; cholesterol 66.3mg; vitamin a iu 1160.7IU; vitamin c 5.6mg; calcium 99.4mg; iron 2.8mg; magnesium 108.6mg; potassium 774.4mg; sodium 707mg.

Beet & Shrimp Winter Salad

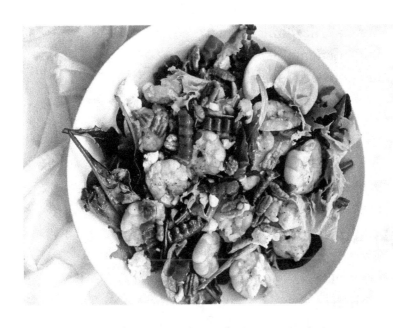

Preparation time:	Serving:
15 minutes	1

Ingredients:
Salad:
- Two cups arugula
- One cup watercress
- One cup cooked beet wedges
- Half cup zucchini ribbons
- Half cup fennel – thinly sliced
- Half cup cooked barley
- 4-ounces shrimp – tails left, cooked, peeled
- Fennel fronds – for garnish

Vinaigrette:
- Two tablespoons extra-virgin olive oil
- One tablespoon red- or white-wine vinegar
- Half teaspoon Dijon mustard
- Half teaspoon minced shallot
- ¼ teaspoon ground pepper
- 1/8 teaspoon salt

Instructions:
- Add shrimp, barley, fennel, zucchini, beets, watercress, and arugula onto the plate.
- Whisk the salt, pepper, shallot, mustard, vinegar, and oil into the bowl. Drizzle over the salad.

Additional Tip:
- Garnish with fennel fronds.

Nutrition:
584 calories; protein 35g; carbohydrates 47g; dietary fiber 9.3g; sugars 17.9g; fat 29.8g; saturated fat 4.2g; cholesterol 214.3mg; vitamin a iu 2645.3IU; vitamin c 43.3mg; calcium 255.5mg; iron 4.3mg; magnesium 147mg; potassium 1506mg; sodium 653.6mg; thiamin 0.2mg.

Farfalle with Tuna, Lemon, and Fennel

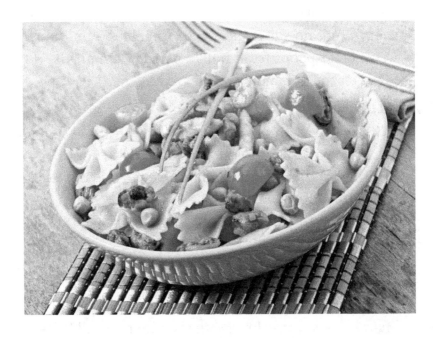

Preparation time:	Serving:
5 minutes	4

Ingredients:

- 6-ounces dried whole grain farfalle pasta
- 5 ounce solid white tuna
- Olive oil – as needed
- One cup fennel – thinly sliced
- Two cloves garlic – minced
- Half teaspoon crushed red pepper
- ¼ teaspoon salt
- 14.5 ounce no-salt-added diced tomatoes – undrained
- Two tablespoons fresh Italian parsley – snipped
- One teaspoon lemon peel – shredded

Instructions:

- First, cook pasta according to packet instruction. Drain it. Place pasta back to the pan. Cover with lid.
- During this, drain tuna and reserve oil. Add olive oil and flake tuna. Keep it aside.
- Add three tbsp reserved oil into a saucepan and cook over a medium flame.
- Add fennel and cook for three minutes. Add salt, crushed red pepper, and garlic and cook for one minute.
- Add in tomatoes and boil it. Decrease the speed of the flame. Let simmer for five to six minutes until thick.
- Add in tuna and simmer for one minute. Add tuna mixture over pasta and stir well.

Additional Tip:

- Sprinkle with lemon peel and parsley.

Nutrition:

356 calories; protein 16.7g; carbohydrates 42.8g; dietary fiber 8.6g; sugars 8.1g; fat 14.2g; saturated fat 1.9g; cholesterol 11mg; vitamin a iu 1060.9IU; vitamin c 20.9mg; calcium 50.9mg; iron 2.3mg; magnesium 62.2mg; potassium 225.5mg; sodium 380.1mg.

Tasty Black Bass with Sautéed Vegetables

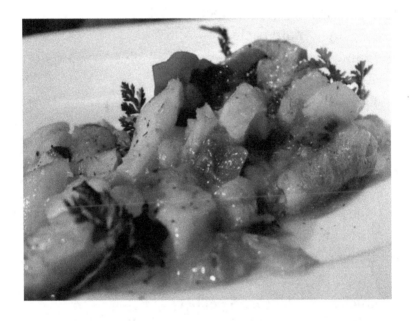

Preparation time:	Cooking time:	Serving:
10 minutes	2 hours and 20 minutes	4

Ingredients:

- One pound raw shrimp, unpeeled, head-on
- Four tablespoons olive oil
- 1/3 cup onion – chopped
- Three cloves garlic – smashed
- One cup fennel – chopped
- Half cup carrot – chopped
- Half cup celery – chopped
- 1/3 cup tomato paste
- Half cup Pernod or other pastis – plus 2 tablespoons
- Eight cups water
- One bay leaf
- Two sprigs fresh thyme
- One teaspoon crushed red pepper
- One teaspoon whole peppercorns
- ¾ teaspoon kosher salt
- One yellow squash – diced
- One zucchini – diced
- 15 cherry tomatoes – halved
- Two tablespoons butter
- One teaspoon ground pepper
- 5-ounce skin-on black bass or cod fillets
- Chopped fennel fronds, fresh tarragon, lemon zest & fennel pollen – for garnish

Instructions:

- Preheat the oven to 350 degrees Fahrenheit.
- Coat the baking pan with cooking spray.
- Cut off the head of the shrimp and place the head on the pan. Pull off and remove legs. Peel and devein the shrimp. Keep the shrimp aside into the fridge and add shells to the pan. Cook the shells and heads for fifteen minutes until crisp.

- During this, add one and a half tbsp oil into the pot and cook over a medium-low flame. Add garlic and onion and cook for five minutes.
- Add fennel, carrot, and celery and cook for eight minutes.
- Add tomato paste and cook and stir for one minute.
- Add half cup Pernod and cook and stir for one minute.
- Add peppercorns, shells, roasted heads, crushed red pepper, thyme, bay leaf, water, and reserved shrimp and boil the mixture over a high flame. Decrease the speed of the flame. Cook for one to one and half hours. Remove the bay leaf.
- Transfer the mixture to the blender and blend until smooth.
- Add through a sieve into the saucepan and press on the solids to get a liquid – season with half tsp salt.
- Add one and half tbsp oil into the skillet and cook over a medium flame.
- Add zucchini and squash and cook for ten to twelve minutes. Add in remaining Pernod and tomatoes and scrape the brown bits. Add in pepper and one tbsp butter.
- Pat dry fish with a paper towel. Sprinkle with salt.
- Add one tbsp oil into the skillet and cook over a medium-high flame.
- Add fish and cook for five minutes. Turnover the fish and add the remaining one tbsp butter. Cook for three to five minutes and baste with butter.
- Split the vegetables between four bowls. Top with fish. Add ¼ cup of cioppino jus.

Additional Tip:

- Garnish with fennel pollen, lemon zest, tarragon, and fennel fronds.

Nutrition:

383 calories; protein 34.7g; carbohydrates 14.7g; dietary fiber 2.5g; sugars 10.8g; fat 18.1g; saturated fat 5.1g; cholesterol 116.6mg; vitamin a iu 2019.8IU; vitamin c 28.5mg; folate 47.6mcg; calcium 69.7mg; iron 1.4mg; magnesium 101.6mg; potassium 973.1mg; sodium 614mg.

CPSIA information can be obtained
at www.ICGtesting.com
Printed in the USA
BVHW091658120521
607126BV00006B/757